WORKOUT LOG

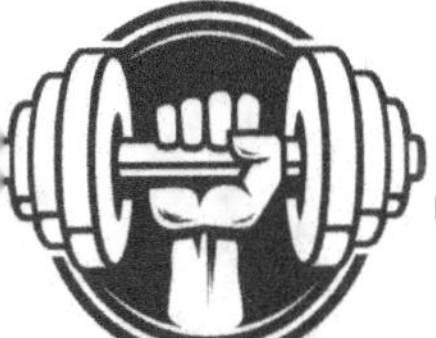

NAME:

GOALS:

DATE:

STATS:

WEIGHT:

I0711648

EXERCISE:	SETS	REPS	WEIGHT	REST	SETS	REPS	WEIGHT	REST	SETS	REPS	WEIGHT	REST	SETS	REPS	WEIGHT	REST

CARDIO:	TIME	DIST.	INT.	PACE	TIME	DIST.	INT.	PACE	TIME	DIST.	INT.	PACE	TIME	DIST.	INT.	PACE

WORKOUT LOG

NAME: ___________________________

GOALS: ___________________________

DATE: ___________________________

STATS: ___________________________

WEIGHT: ___________________________

EXERCISE:	SETS	REPS	WEIGHT	REST	SETS	REPS	WEIGHT	REST	SETS	REPS	WEIGHT	REST	SETS	REPS	WEIGHT	REST

CARDIO:	TIME	DIST.	INT.	PACE	TIME	DIST.	INT.	PACE	TIME	DIST.	INT.	PACE	TIME	DIST.	INT.	PACE

WORKOUT LOG

NAME:
GOALS:
DATE:
STATS:
WEIGHT:

EXERCISE:	SETS	REPS	WEIGHT	REST	SETS	REPS	WEIGHT	REST	SETS	REPS	WEIGHT	REST	SETS	REPS	WEIGHT	REST

CARDIO:	TIME	DIST.	INT.	PACE	TIME	DIST.	INT.	PACE	TIME	DIST.	INT.	PACE	TIME	DIST.	INT.	PACE

WORKOUT LOG

NAME:

GOALS:

DATE:

STATS:

WEIGHT:

EXERCISE:	SETS	REPS	WEIGHT	REST	SETS	REPS	WEIGHT	REST	SETS	REPS	WEIGHT	REST	SETS	REPS	WEIGHT	REST

CARDIO:	TIME	DIST.	INT.	PACE	TIME	DIST.	INT.	PACE	TIME	DIST.	INT.	PACE	TIME	DIST.	INT.	PACE

WORKOUT LOG

NAME: ________________________

GOALS: ________________________

DATE:

STATS:

WEIGHT:

EXERCISE:	SETS	REPS	WEIGHT	REST	SETS	REPS	WEIGHT	REST	SETS	REPS	WEIGHT	REST	SETS	REPS	WEIGHT	REST

CARDIO:	TIME	DIST.	INT.	PACE	TIME	DIST.	INT.	PACE	TIME	DIST.	INT.	PACE	TIME	DIST.	INT.	PACE

WORKOUT LOG

NAME:
GOALS:
DATE:
STATS:
WEIGHT:

EXERCISE:	SETS	REPS	WEIGHT	REST	SETS	REPS	WEIGHT	REST	SETS	REPS	WEIGHT	REST	SETS	REPS	WEIGHT	REST

CARDIO:	TIME	DIST.	INT.	PACE	TIME	DIST.	INT.	PACE	TIME	DIST.	INT.	PACE	TIME	DIST.	INT.	PACE

WORKOUT LOG

NAME:
GOALS:
DATE:
STATS:
WEIGHT:

EXERCISE:	SETS	REPS	WEIGHT	REST	SETS	REPS	WEIGHT	REST	SETS	REPS	WEIGHT	REST	SETS	REPS	WEIGHT	REST

CARDIO:	TIME	DIST.	INT.	PACE	TIME	DIST.	INT.	PACE	TIME	DIST.	INT.	PACE	TIME	DIST.	INT.	PACE

WORKOUT LOG

NAME:
GOALS:
DATE:
STATS:
WEIGHT:

EXERCISE:	SETS	REPS	WEIGHT	REST	SETS	REPS	WEIGHT	REST	SETS	REPS	WEIGHT	REST	SETS	REPS	WEIGHT	REST

CARDIO:	TIME	DIST.	INT.	PACE	TIME	DIST.	INT.	PACE	TIME	DIST.	INT.	PACE	TIME	DIST.	INT.	PACE

WORKOUT LOG

NAME:
GOALS:
DATE:
STATS:
WEIGHT:

EXERCISE:	SETS	REPS	WEIGHT	REST	SETS	REPS	WEIGHT	REST	SETS	REPS	WEIGHT	REST	SETS	REPS	WEIGHT	REST

CARDIO:	TIME	DIST.	INT.	PACE	TIME	DIST.	INT.	PACE	TIME	DIST.	INT.	PACE	TIME	DIST.	INT.	PACE

WORKOUT LOG

NAME:

GOALS:

DATE:

STATS:

WEIGHT:

EXERCISE:	SETS	REPS	WEIGHT	REST	SETS	REPS	WEIGHT	REST	SETS	REPS	WEIGHT	REST	SETS	REPS	WEIGHT	REST

CARDIO:	TIME	DIST.	INT.	PACE	TIME	DIST.	INT.	PACE	TIME	DIST.	INT.	PACE	TIME	DIST.	INT.	PACE

WORKOUT LOG

NAME: ______________________
GOALS: ______________________
DATE:
STATS:
WEIGHT:

EXERCISE:	SETS	REPS	WEIGHT	REST	SETS	REPS	WEIGHT	REST	SETS	REPS	WEIGHT	REST	SETS	REPS	WEIGHT	REST

CARDIO:	TIME	DIST.	INT.	PACE	TIME	DIST.	INT.	PACE	TIME	DIST.	INT.	PACE	TIME	DIST.	INT.	PACE

WORKOUT LOG

NAME:

GOALS:

DATE:

STATS:

WEIGHT:

EXERCISE:	SETS	REPS	WEIGHT	REST	SETS	REPS	WEIGHT	REST	SETS	REPS	WEIGHT	REST	SETS	REPS	WEIGHT	REST

CARDIO:	TIME	DIST.	INT.	PACE	TIME	DIST.	INT.	PACE	TIME	DIST.	INT.	PACE	TIME	DIST.	INT.	PACE

WORKOUT LOG

NAME:

GOALS:

DATE:

STATS:

WEIGHT:

EXERCISE:	SETS	REPS	WEIGHT	REST	SETS	REPS	WEIGHT	REST	SETS	REPS	WEIGHT	REST	SETS	REPS	WEIGHT	REST

CARDIO:	TIME	DIST.	INT.	PACE	TIME	DIST.	INT.	PACE	TIME	DIST.	INT.	PACE	TIME	DIST.	INT.	PACE

WORKOUT LOG

NAME:

GOALS:

DATE:

STATS:

WEIGHT:

EXERCISE:	SETS	REPS	WEIGHT	REST	SETS	REPS	WEIGHT	REST	SETS	REPS	WEIGHT	REST	SETS	REPS	WEIGHT	REST

CARDIO:	TIME	DIST.	INT.	PACE	TIME	DIST.	INT.	PACE	TIME	DIST.	INT.	PACE	TIME	DIST.	INT.	PACE

WORKOUT LOG

NAME:

GOALS:

DATE:

STATS:

WEIGHT:

EXERCISE:	SETS	REPS	WEIGHT	REST	SETS	REPS	WEIGHT	REST	SETS	REPS	WEIGHT	REST	SETS	REPS	WEIGHT	REST

CARDIO:	TIME	DIST.	INT.	PACE	TIME	DIST.	INT.	PACE	TIME	DIST.	INT.	PACE	TIME	DIST.	INT.	PACE

WORKOUT LOG

NAME: _______________________________________

GOALS: _______________________________________

DATE:

STATS:

WEIGHT:

EXERCISE:	SETS	REPS	WEIGHT	REST	SETS	REPS	WEIGHT	REST	SETS	REPS	WEIGHT	REST	SETS	REPS	WEIGHT	REST

CARDIO:	TIME	DIST.	INT.	PACE	TIME	DIST.	INT.	PACE	TIME	DIST.	INT.	PACE	TIME	DIST.	INT.	PACE

WORKOUT LOG

NAME:

GOALS:

DATE:

STATS:

WEIGHT:

EXERCISE:	SETS	REPS	WEIGHT	REST	SETS	REPS	WEIGHT	REST	SETS	REPS	WEIGHT	REST	SETS	REPS	WEIGHT	REST

CARDIO:	TIME	DIST.	INT.	PACE	TIME	DIST.	INT.	PACE	TIME	DIST.	INT.	PACE	TIME	DIST.	INT.	PACE

WORKOUT LOG

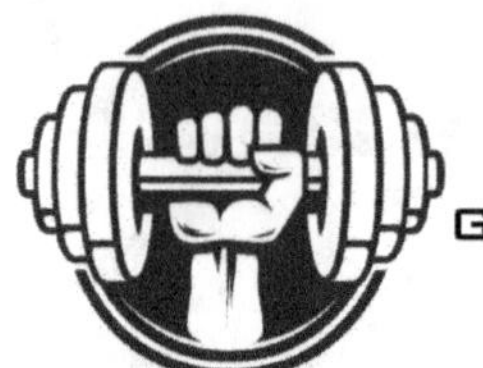

NAME:

GOALS:

DATE:

STATS:

WEIGHT:

EXERCISE:	SETS	REPS	WEIGHT	REST	SETS	REPS	WEIGHT	REST	SETS	REPS	WEIGHT	REST	SETS	REPS	WEIGHT	REST

CARDIO:	TIME	DIST.	INT.	PACE	TIME	DIST.	INT.	PACE	TIME	DIST.	INT.	PACE	TIME	DIST.	INT.	PACE

WORKOUT LOG

NAME:
GOALS:
DATE:
STATS:
WEIGHT:

EXERCISE:	SETS	REPS	WEIGHT	REST	SETS	REPS	WEIGHT	REST	SETS	REPS	WEIGHT	REST	SETS	REPS	WEIGHT	REST

CARDIO:	TIME	DIST.	INT.	PACE	TIME	DIST.	INT.	PACE	TIME	DIST.	INT.	PACE	TIME	DIST.	INT.	PACE

WORKOUT LOG

NAME:
GOALS:
DATE:
STATS:
WEIGHT:

EXERCISE:	SETS	REPS	WEIGHT	REST	SETS	REPS	WEIGHT	REST	SETS	REPS	WEIGHT	REST	SETS	REPS	WEIGHT	REST

CARDIO:	TIME	DIST.	INT.	PACE	TIME	DIST.	INT.	PACE	TIME	DIST.	INT.	PACE	TIME	DIST.	INT.	PACE

WORKOUT LOG

NAME:
GOALS:
DATE:
STATS:
WEIGHT:

EXERCISE:	SETS	REPS	WEIGHT	REST	SETS	REPS	WEIGHT	REST	SETS	REPS	WEIGHT	REST	SETS	REPS	WEIGHT	REST

CARDIO:	TIME	DIST.	INT.	PACE	TIME	DIST.	INT.	PACE	TIME	DIST.	INT.	PACE	TIME	DIST.	INT.	PACE

WORKOUT LOG

NAME:
GOALS:
DATE:
STATS:
WEIGHT:

EXERCISE:	SETS	REPS	WEIGHT	REST	SETS	REPS	WEIGHT	REST	SETS	REPS	WEIGHT	REST	SETS	REPS	WEIGHT	REST

CARDIO:	TIME	DIST.	INT.	PACE	TIME	DIST.	INT.	PACE	TIME	DIST.	INT.	PACE	TIME	DIST.	INT.	PACE

WORKOUT LOG

NAME: _______________________

GOALS: _______________________

DATE:

STATS:

WEIGHT:

EXERCISE:	SETS	REPS	WEIGHT	REST	SETS	REPS	WEIGHT	REST	SETS	REPS	WEIGHT	REST	SETS	REPS	WEIGHT	REST

CARDIO:	TIME	DIST.	INT.	PACE	TIME	DIST.	INT.	PACE	TIME	DIST.	INT.	PACE	TIME	DIST.	INT.	PACE

WORKOUT LOG

NAME:

GOALS:

DATE:

STATS:

WEIGHT:

EXERCISE:	SETS	REPS	WEIGHT	REST	SETS	REPS	WEIGHT	REST	SETS	REPS	WEIGHT	REST	SETS	REPS	WEIGHT	REST

CARDIO:	TIME	DIST.	INT.	PACE	TIME	DIST.	INT.	PACE	TIME	DIST.	INT.	PACE	TIME	DIST.	INT.	PACE

WORKOUT LOG

NAME:
GOALS:
DATE:
STATS:
WEIGHT:

EXERCISE:	SETS	REPS	WEIGHT	REST	SETS	REPS	WEIGHT	REST	SETS	REPS	WEIGHT	REST	SETS	REPS	WEIGHT	REST

CARDIO:	TIME	DIST.	INT.	PACE	TIME	DIST.	INT.	PACE	TIME	DIST.	INT.	PACE	TIME	DIST.	INT.	PACE

WORKOUT LOG

NAME:

GOALS:

DATE:

STATS:

WEIGHT:

EXERCISE:	SETS	REPS	WEIGHT	REST	SETS	REPS	WEIGHT	REST	SETS	REPS	WEIGHT	REST	SETS	REPS	WEIGHT	REST

CARDIO:	TIME	DIST.	INT.	PACE	TIME	DIST.	INT.	PACE	TIME	DIST.	INT.	PACE	TIME	DIST.	INT.	PACE

WORKOUT LOG

NAME:

GOALS:

DATE:

STATS:

WEIGHT:

EXERCISE:	SETS	REPS	WEIGHT	REST	SETS	REPS	WEIGHT	REST	SETS	REPS	WEIGHT	REST	SETS	REPS	WEIGHT	REST

CARDIO:	TIME	DIST.	INT.	PACE	TIME	DIST.	INT.	PACE	TIME	DIST.	INT.	PACE	TIME	DIST.	INT.	PACE

WORKOUT LOG

NAME:

GOALS:

DATE:

STATS:

WEIGHT:

EXERCISE:	SETS	REPS	WEIGHT	REST	SETS	REPS	WEIGHT	REST	SETS	REPS	WEIGHT	REST	SETS	REPS	WEIGHT	REST

CARDIO:	TIME	DIST.	INT.	PACE	TIME	DIST.	INT.	PACE	TIME	DIST.	INT.	PACE	TIME	DIST.	INT.	PACE

WORKOUT LOG

NAME:

GOALS:

DATE:

STATS:

WEIGHT:

EXERCISE:	SETS	REPS	WEIGHT	REST	SETS	REPS	WEIGHT	REST	SETS	REPS	WEIGHT	REST	SETS	REPS	WEIGHT	REST

CARDIO:	TIME	DIST.	INT.	PACE	TIME	DIST.	INT.	PACE	TIME	DIST.	INT.	PACE	TIME	DIST.	INT.	PACE

WORKOUT LOG

NAME:
GOALS:
DATE:
STATS:
WEIGHT:

EXERCISE:	SETS	REPS	WEIGHT	REST	SETS	REPS	WEIGHT	REST	SETS	REPS	WEIGHT	REST	SETS	REPS	WEIGHT	REST

CARDIO:	TIME	DIST.	INT.	PACE	TIME	DIST.	INT.	PACE	TIME	DIST.	INT.	PACE	TIME	DIST.	INT.	PACE

WORKOUT LOG

NAME:

GOALS:

DATE:

STATS:

WEIGHT:

EXERCISE:	SETS	REPS	WEIGHT	REST	SETS	REPS	WEIGHT	REST	SETS	REPS	WEIGHT	REST	SETS	REPS	WEIGHT	REST

CARDIO:	TIME	DIST.	INT.	PACE	TIME	DIST.	INT.	PACE	TIME	DIST.	INT.	PACE	TIME	DIST.	INT.	PACE

WORKOUT LOG

NAME:
GOALS:
DATE:
STATS:
WEIGHT:

EXERCISE:	SETS	REPS	WEIGHT	REST	SETS	REPS	WEIGHT	REST	SETS	REPS	WEIGHT	REST	SETS	REPS	WEIGHT	REST

CARDIO:	TIME	DIST.	INT.	PACE	TIME	DIST.	INT.	PACE	TIME	DIST.	INT.	PACE	TIME	DIST.	INT.	PACE

WORKOUT LOG

NAME:
GOALS:
DATE:
STATS:
WEIGHT:

EXERCISE:	SETS	REPS	WEIGHT	REST	SETS	REPS	WEIGHT	REST	SETS	REPS	WEIGHT	REST	SETS	REPS	WEIGHT	REST

CARDIO:	TIME	DIST.	INT.	PACE	TIME	DIST.	INT.	PACE	TIME	DIST.	INT.	PACE	TIME	DIST.	INT.	PACE

WORKOUT LOG

NAME: _______________

GOALS: _______________

DATE:

STATS:

WEIGHT:

EXERCISE:	SETS	REPS	WEIGHT	REST	SETS	REPS	WEIGHT	REST	SETS	REPS	WEIGHT	REST	SETS	REPS	WEIGHT	REST

CARDIO:	TIME	DIST.	INT.	PACE	TIME	DIST.	INT.	PACE	TIME	DIST.	INT.	PACE	TIME	DIST.	INT.	PACE

WORKOUT LOG

NAME:
GOALS:
DATE:
STATS:
WEIGHT:

EXERCISE:	SETS	REPS	WEIGHT	REST	SETS	REPS	WEIGHT	REST	SETS	REPS	WEIGHT	REST	SETS	REPS	WEIGHT	REST

CARDIO:	TIME	DIST.	INT.	PACE	TIME	DIST.	INT.	PACE	TIME	DIST.	INT.	PACE	TIME	DIST.	INT.	PACE

WORKOUT LOG

NAME:
GOALS:
DATE:
STATS:
WEIGHT:

EXERCISE:	SETS	REPS	WEIGHT	REST	SETS	REPS	WEIGHT	REST	SETS	REPS	WEIGHT	REST	SETS	REPS	WEIGHT	REST

CARDIO:	TIME	DIST.	INT.	PACE	TIME	DIST.	INT.	PACE	TIME	DIST.	INT.	PACE	TIME	DIST.	INT.	PACE

WORKOUT LOG

NAME:
GOALS:
DATE:
STATS:
WEIGHT:

EXERCISE:	SETS	REPS	WEIGHT	REST	SETS	REPS	WEIGHT	REST	SETS	REPS	WEIGHT	REST	SETS	REPS	WEIGHT	REST

CARDIO:	TIME	DIST.	INT.	PACE	TIME	DIST.	INT.	PACE	TIME	DIST.	INT.	PACE	TIME	DIST.	INT.	PACE

WORKOUT LOG

NAME:
GOALS:
DATE:
STATS:
WEIGHT:

EXERCISE:	SETS	REPS	WEIGHT	REST	SETS	REPS	WEIGHT	REST	SETS	REPS	WEIGHT	REST	SETS	REPS	WEIGHT	REST

CARDIO:	TIME	DIST.	INT.	PACE	TIME	DIST.	INT.	PACE	TIME	DIST.	INT.	PACE	TIME	DIST.	INT.	PACE

WORKOUT LOG

NAME:

GOALS:

DATE:

STATS:

WEIGHT:

EXERCISE:	SETS	REPS	WEIGHT	REST	SETS	REPS	WEIGHT	REST	SETS	REPS	WEIGHT	REST	SETS	REPS	WEIGHT	REST

CARDIO:	TIME	DIST.	INT.	PACE	TIME	DIST.	INT.	PACE	TIME	DIST.	INT.	PACE	TIME	DIST.	INT.	PACE

WORKOUT LOG

NAME:
GOALS:
DATE:
STATS:
WEIGHT:

EXERCISE:	SETS	REPS	WEIGHT	REST	SETS	REPS	WEIGHT	REST	SETS	REPS	WEIGHT	REST	SETS	REPS	WEIGHT	REST

CARDIO:	TIME	DIST.	INT.	PACE	TIME	DIST.	INT.	PACE	TIME	DIST.	INT.	PACE	TIME	DIST.	INT.	PACE

WORKOUT LOG

NAME:
GOALS:
DATE:
STATS:
WEIGHT:

EXERCISE:	SETS	REPS	WEIGHT	REST	SETS	REPS	WEIGHT	REST	SETS	REPS	WEIGHT	REST	SETS	REPS	WEIGHT	REST

CARDIO:	TIME	DIST.	INT.	PACE	TIME	DIST.	INT.	PACE	TIME	DIST.	INT.	PACE	TIME	DIST.	INT.	PACE

WORKOUT LOG

NAME: ________________________________

GOALS: ________________________________

DATE:

STATS:

WEIGHT:

EXERCISE:	SETS	REPS	WEIGHT	REST	SETS	REPS	WEIGHT	REST	SETS	REPS	WEIGHT	REST	SETS	REPS	WEIGHT	REST

CARDIO:	TIME	DIST.	INT.	PACE	TIME	DIST.	INT.	PACE	TIME	DIST.	INT.	PACE	TIME	DIST.	INT.	PACE

WORKOUT LOG

NAME:

GOALS:

DATE:

STATS:

WEIGHT:

EXERCISE:	SETS	REPS	WEIGHT	REST	SETS	REPS	WEIGHT	REST	SETS	REPS	WEIGHT	REST	SETS	REPS	WEIGHT	REST

CARDIO:	TIME	DIST.	INT.	PACE	TIME	DIST.	INT.	PACE	TIME	DIST.	INT.	PACE	TIME	DIST.	INT.	PACE

WORKOUT LOG

NAME:

GOALS:

DATE:

STATS:

WEIGHT:

EXERCISE:	SETS	REPS	WEIGHT	REST	SETS	REPS	WEIGHT	REST	SETS	REPS	WEIGHT	REST	SETS	REPS	WEIGHT	REST

CARDIO:	TIME	DIST.	INT.	PACE	TIME	DIST.	INT.	PACE	TIME	DIST.	INT.	PACE	TIME	DIST.	INT.	PACE

WORKOUT LOG

NAME: ____________________

GOALS: ____________________

DATE:

STATS:

WEIGHT:

EXERCISE:	SETS	REPS	WEIGHT	REST	SETS	REPS	WEIGHT	REST	SETS	REPS	WEIGHT	REST	SETS	REPS	WEIGHT	REST

CARDIO:	TIME	DIST.	INT.	PACE	TIME	DIST.	INT.	PACE	TIME	DIST.	INT.	PACE	TIME	DIST.	INT.	PACE

WORKOUT LOG

NAME:
GOALS:
DATE:
STATS:
WEIGHT:

EXERCISE:	SETS	REPS	WEIGHT	REST	SETS	REPS	WEIGHT	REST	SETS	REPS	WEIGHT	REST	SETS	REPS	WEIGHT	REST

CARDIO:	TIME	DIST.	INT.	PACE	TIME	DIST.	INT.	PACE	TIME	DIST.	INT.	PACE	TIME	DIST.	INT.	PACE

WORKOUT LOG

NAME:
GOALS:
DATE:
STATS:
WEIGHT:

EXERCISE:	SETS	REPS	WEIGHT	REST	SETS	REPS	WEIGHT	REST	SETS	REPS	WEIGHT	REST	SETS	REPS	WEIGHT	REST

CARDIO:	TIME	DIST.	INT.	PACE	TIME	DIST.	INT.	PACE	TIME	DIST.	INT.	PACE	TIME	DIST.	INT.	PACE

WORKOUT LOG

NAME:
GOALS:
DATE:
STATS:
WEIGHT:

EXERCISE:	SETS	REPS	WEIGHT	REST	SETS	REPS	WEIGHT	REST	SETS	REPS	WEIGHT	REST	SETS	REPS	WEIGHT	REST

CARDIO:	TIME	DIST.	INT.	PACE	TIME	DIST.	INT.	PACE	TIME	DIST.	INT.	PACE	TIME	DIST.	INT.	PACE

WORKOUT LOG

NAME:
GOALS:
DATE:
STATS:
WEIGHT:

EXERCISE:	SETS	REPS	WEIGHT	REST	SETS	REPS	WEIGHT	REST	SETS	REPS	WEIGHT	REST	SETS	REPS	WEIGHT	REST

CARDIO:	TIME	DIST.	INT.	PACE	TIME	DIST.	INT.	PACE	TIME	DIST.	INT.	PACE	TIME	DIST.	INT.	PACE

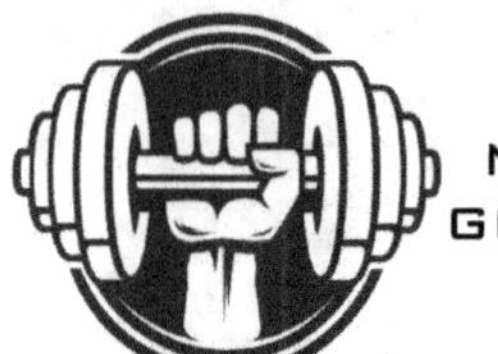

WORKOUT LOG

NAME: ___________________________

GOALS: ___________________________

DATE: ___________________________

STATS: ___________________________

WEIGHT: ___________________________

EXERCISE:	SETS	REPS	WEIGHT	REST	SETS	REPS	WEIGHT	REST	SETS	REPS	WEIGHT	REST	SETS	REPS	WEIGHT	REST

CARDIO:	TIME	DIST.	INT.	PACE	TIME	DIST.	INT.	PACE	TIME	DIST.	INT.	PACE	TIME	DIST.	INT.	PACE

WORKOUT LOG

NAME:

GOALS:

DATE:

STATS:

WEIGHT:

EXERCISE:	SETS	REPS	WEIGHT	REST	SETS	REPS	WEIGHT	REST	SETS	REPS	WEIGHT	REST	SETS	REPS	WEIGHT	REST

CARDIO:	TIME	DIST.	INT.	PACE	TIME	DIST.	INT.	PACE	TIME	DIST.	INT.	PACE	TIME	DIST.	INT.	PACE

WORKOUT LOG

NAME:
GOALS:
DATE:
STATS:
WEIGHT:

EXERCISE:	SETS	REPS	WEIGHT	REST	SETS	REPS	WEIGHT	REST	SETS	REPS	WEIGHT	REST	SETS	REPS	WEIGHT	REST

CARDIO:	TIME	DIST.	INT.	PACE	TIME	DIST.	INT.	PACE	TIME	DIST.	INT.	PACE	TIME	DIST.	INT.	PACE

WORKOUT LOG

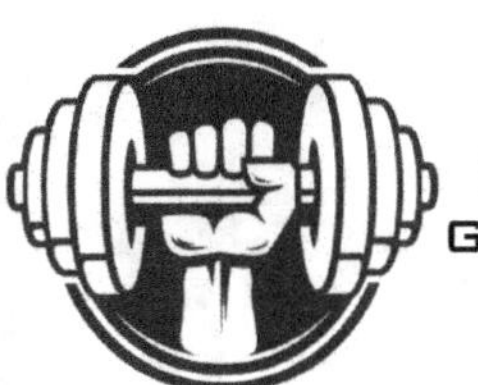

NAME:

GOALS:

DATE:

STATS:

WEIGHT:

EXERCISE:	SETS	REPS	WEIGHT	REST	SETS	REPS	WEIGHT	REST	SETS	REPS	WEIGHT	REST	SETS	REPS	WEIGHT	REST

CARDIO:	TIME	DIST.	INT.	PACE	TIME	DIST.	INT.	PACE	TIME	DIST.	INT.	PACE	TIME	DIST.	INT.	PACE

WORKOUT LOG

NAME: ___________________________

GOALS: ___________________________

DATE:

STATS:

WEIGHT:

EXERCISE:	SETS	REPS	WEIGHT	REST	SETS	REPS	WEIGHT	REST	SETS	REPS	WEIGHT	REST	SETS	REPS	WEIGHT	REST

CARDIO:	TIME	DIST.	INT.	PACE	TIME	DIST.	INT.	PACE	TIME	DIST.	INT.	PACE	TIME	DIST.	INT.	PACE

WORKOUT LOG

NAME:
GOALS:
DATE:
STATS:
WEIGHT:

EXERCISE:	SETS	REPS	WEIGHT	REST	SETS	REPS	WEIGHT	REST	SETS	REPS	WEIGHT	REST	SETS	REPS	WEIGHT	REST

CARDIO:	TIME	DIST.	INT.	PACE	TIME	DIST.	INT.	PACE	TIME	DIST.	INT.	PACE	TIME	DIST.	INT.	PACE

WORKOUT LOG

NAME: _______________________________________

GOALS: ______________________________________

DATE:

STATS:

WEIGHT:

EXERCISE:	SETS	REPS	WEIGHT	REST	SETS	REPS	WEIGHT	REST	SETS	REPS	WEIGHT	REST	SETS	REPS	WEIGHT	REST

CARDIO:	TIME	DIST.	INT.	PACE	TIME	DIST.	INT.	PACE	TIME	DIST.	INT.	PACE	TIME	DIST.	INT.	PACE

WORKOUT LOG

NAME: ____

GOALS: ____

DATE:

STATS:

WEIGHT:

EXERCISE:	SETS	REPS	WEIGHT	REST	SETS	REPS	WEIGHT	REST	SETS	REPS	WEIGHT	REST	SETS	REPS	WEIGHT	REST

CARDIO:	TIME	DIST.	INT.	PACE	TIME	DIST.	INT.	PACE	TIME	DIST.	INT.	PACE	TIME	DIST.	INT.	PACE

WORKOUT LOG

NAME: _______________________

GOALS: _______________________

DATE:

STATS:

WEIGHT:

EXERCISE:	SETS	REPS	WEIGHT	REST	SETS	REPS	WEIGHT	REST	SETS	REPS	WEIGHT	REST	SETS	REPS	WEIGHT	REST

CARDIO:	TIME	DIST.	INT.	PACE	TIME	DIST.	INT.	PACE	TIME	DIST.	INT.	PACE	TIME	DIST.	INT.	PACE

WORKOUT LOG

NAME: __________________________________

GOALS: _________________________________

DATE:

STATS:

WEIGHT:

EXERCISE:	SETS	REPS	WEIGHT	REST	SETS	REPS	WEIGHT	REST	SETS	REPS	WEIGHT	REST	SETS	REPS	WEIGHT	REST

CARDIO:	TIME	DIST.	INT.	PACE	TIME	DIST.	INT.	PACE	TIME	DIST.	INT.	PACE	TIME	DIST.	INT.	PACE

WORKOUT LOG

NAME:

GOALS:

DATE:

STATS:

WEIGHT:

EXERCISE:	SETS	REPS	WEIGHT	REST	SETS	REPS	WEIGHT	REST	SETS	REPS	WEIGHT	REST	SETS	REPS	WEIGHT	REST

CARDIO:	TIME	DIST.	INT.	PACE	TIME	DIST.	INT.	PACE	TIME	DIST.	INT.	PACE	TIME	DIST.	INT.	PACE

WORKOUT LOG

NAME:
GOALS:
DATE:
STATS:
WEIGHT:

EXERCISE:	SETS	REPS	WEIGHT	REST	SETS	REPS	WEIGHT	REST	SETS	REPS	WEIGHT	REST	SETS	REPS	WEIGHT	REST

CARDIO:	TIME	DIST.	INT.	PACE	TIME	DIST.	INT.	PACE	TIME	DIST.	INT.	PACE	TIME	DIST.	INT.	PACE

WORKOUT LOG

NAME:

GOALS:

DATE:

STATS:

WEIGHT:

EXERCISE:	SETS	REPS	WEIGHT	REST	SETS	REPS	WEIGHT	REST	SETS	REPS	WEIGHT	REST	SETS	REPS	WEIGHT	REST

CARDIO:	TIME	DIST.	INT.	PACE	TIME	DIST.	INT.	PACE	TIME	DIST.	INT.	PACE	TIME	DIST.	INT.	PACE

WORKOUT LOG

NAME: ___________________________________

GOALS: ___________________________________

DATE:

STATS:

WEIGHT:

EXERCISE:	SETS	REPS	WEIGHT	REST	SETS	REPS	WEIGHT	REST	SETS	REPS	WEIGHT	REST	SETS	REPS	WEIGHT	REST

CARDIO:	TIME	DIST.	INT.	PACE	TIME	DIST.	INT.	PACE	TIME	DIST.	INT.	PACE	TIME	DIST.	INT.	PACE

WORKOUT LOG

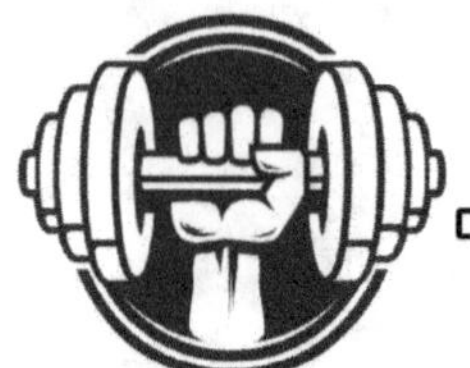

NAME: ________________________

GOALS: ________________________

DATE:

STATS:

WEIGHT:

EXERCISE:	SETS	REPS	WEIGHT	REST	SETS	REPS	WEIGHT	REST	SETS	REPS	WEIGHT	REST	SETS	REPS	WEIGHT	REST

CARDIO:	TIME	DIST.	INT.	PACE	TIME	DIST.	INT.	PACE	TIME	DIST.	INT.	PACE	TIME	DIST.	INT.	PACE

WORKOUT LOG

NAME:

GOALS:

DATE:

STATS:

WEIGHT:

EXERCISE:	SETS	REPS	WEIGHT	REST	SETS	REPS	WEIGHT	REST	SETS	REPS	WEIGHT	REST	SETS	REPS	WEIGHT	REST

CARDIO:	TIME	DIST.	INT.	PACE	TIME	DIST.	INT.	PACE	TIME	DIST.	INT.	PACE	TIME	DIST.	INT.	PACE

WORKOUT LOG

NAME:
GOALS:
DATE:
STATS:
WEIGHT:

EXERCISE:	SETS	REPS	WEIGHT	REST	SETS	REPS	WEIGHT	REST	SETS	REPS	WEIGHT	REST	SETS	REPS	WEIGHT	REST

CARDIO:	TIME	DIST.	INT.	PACE	TIME	DIST.	INT.	PACE	TIME	DIST.	INT.	PACE	TIME	DIST.	INT.	PACE

WORKOUT LOG

NAME:
GOALS:
DATE:
STATS:
WEIGHT:

EXERCISE:	SETS	REPS	WEIGHT	REST	SETS	REPS	WEIGHT	REST	SETS	REPS	WEIGHT	REST	SETS	REPS	WEIGHT	REST

CARDIO:	TIME	DIST.	INT.	PACE	TIME	DIST.	INT.	PACE	TIME	DIST.	INT.	PACE	TIME	DIST.	INT.	PACE

WORKOUT LOG

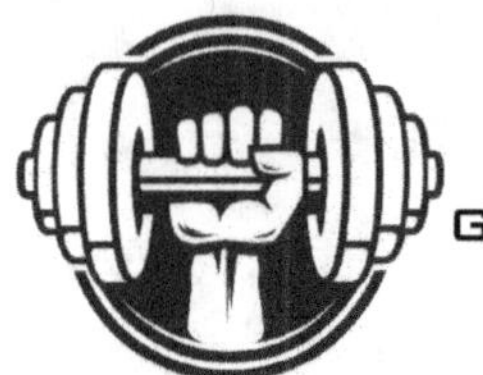

NAME:

GOALS:

DATE:

STATS:

WEIGHT:

EXERCISE:	SETS	REPS	WEIGHT	REST	SETS	REPS	WEIGHT	REST	SETS	REPS	WEIGHT	REST	SETS	REPS	WEIGHT	REST

CARDIO:	TIME	DIST.	INT.	PACE	TIME	DIST.	INT.	PACE	TIME	DIST.	INT.	PACE	TIME	DIST.	INT.	PACE

WORKOUT LOG

NAME:
GOALS:
DATE:
STATS:
WEIGHT:

EXERCISE:	SETS	REPS	WEIGHT	REST	SETS	REPS	WEIGHT	REST	SETS	REPS	WEIGHT	REST	SETS	REPS	WEIGHT	REST

CARDIO:	TIME	DIST.	INT.	PACE	TIME	DIST.	INT.	PACE	TIME	DIST.	INT.	PACE	TIME	DIST.	INT.	PACE

WORKOUT LOG

NAME:
GOALS:
DATE:
STATS:
WEIGHT:

EXERCISE:	SETS	REPS	WEIGHT	REST	SETS	REPS	WEIGHT	REST	SETS	REPS	WEIGHT	REST	SETS	REPS	WEIGHT	REST

CARDIO:	TIME	DIST.	INT.	PACE	TIME	DIST.	INT.	PACE	TIME	DIST.	INT.	PACE	TIME	DIST.	INT.	PACE

WORKOUT LOG

NAME:
GOALS:
DATE:
STATS:
WEIGHT:

EXERCISE:	SETS	REPS	WEIGHT	REST	SETS	REPS	WEIGHT	REST	SETS	REPS	WEIGHT	REST	SETS	REPS	WEIGHT	REST

CARDIO:	TIME	DIST.	INT.	PACE	TIME	DIST.	INT.	PACE	TIME	DIST.	INT.	PACE	TIME	DIST.	INT.	PACE

WORKOUT LOG

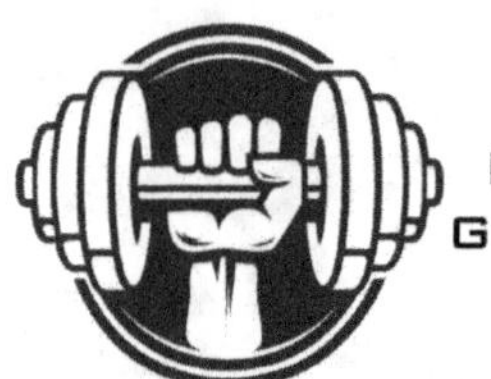

NAME:

GOALS:

DATE:

STATS:

WEIGHT:

EXERCISE:	SETS	REPS	WEIGHT	REST	SETS	REPS	WEIGHT	REST	SETS	REPS	WEIGHT	REST	SETS	REPS	WEIGHT	REST

CARDIO:	TIME	DIST.	INT.	PACE	TIME	DIST.	INT.	PACE	TIME	DIST.	INT.	PACE	TIME	DIST.	INT.	PACE

WORKOUT LOG

NAME:
GOALS:
DATE:
STATS:
WEIGHT:

EXERCISE:	SETS	REPS	WEIGHT	REST	SETS	REPS	WEIGHT	REST	SETS	REPS	WEIGHT	REST	SETS	REPS	WEIGHT	REST

CARDIO:	TIME	DIST.	INT.	PACE	TIME	DIST.	INT.	PACE	TIME	DIST.	INT.	PACE	TIME	DIST.	INT.	PACE

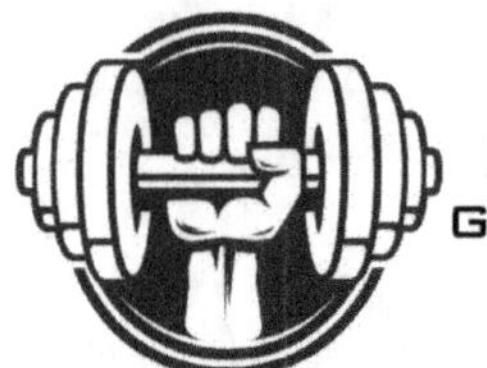

WORKOUT LOG

NAME:
GOALS:
DATE:
STATS:
WEIGHT:

EXERCISE:	SETS	REPS	WEIGHT	REST	SETS	REPS	WEIGHT	REST	SETS	REPS	WEIGHT	REST	SETS	REPS	WEIGHT	REST

CARDIO:	TIME	DIST.	INT.	PACE	TIME	DIST.	INT.	PACE	TIME	DIST.	INT.	PACE	TIME	DIST.	INT.	PACE

WORKOUT LOG

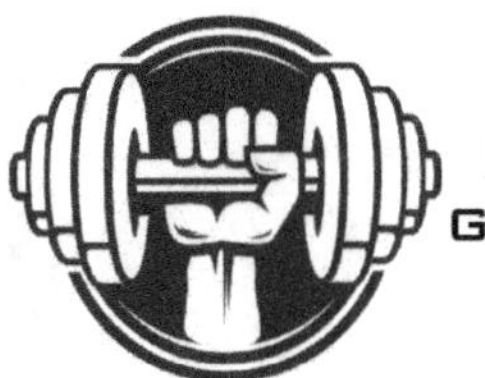

NAME: _______________________________________

GOALS: _______________________________________

DATE:

STATS:

WEIGHT:

EXERCISE:	SETS	REPS	WEIGHT	REST	SETS	REPS	WEIGHT	REST	SETS	REPS	WEIGHT	REST	SETS	REPS	WEIGHT	REST

CARDIO:	TIME	DIST.	INT.	PACE	TIME	DIST.	INT.	PACE	TIME	DIST.	INT.	PACE	TIME	DIST.	INT.	PACE

WORKOUT LOG

NAME:

GOALS:

DATE:

STATS:

WEIGHT:

EXERCISE:	SETS	REPS	WEIGHT	REST	SETS	REPS	WEIGHT	REST	SETS	REPS	WEIGHT	REST	SETS	REPS	WEIGHT	REST

CARDIO:	TIME	DIST.	INT.	PACE	TIME	DIST.	INT.	PACE	TIME	DIST.	INT.	PACE	TIME	DIST.	INT.	PACE

WORKOUT LOG

NAME:

GOALS:

DATE:

STATS:

WEIGHT:

EXERCISE:	SETS	REPS	WEIGHT	REST	SETS	REPS	WEIGHT	REST	SETS	REPS	WEIGHT	REST	SETS	REPS	WEIGHT	REST

CARDIO:	TIME	DIST.	INT.	PACE	TIME	DIST.	INT.	PACE	TIME	DIST.	INT.	PACE	TIME	DIST.	INT.	PACE

WORKOUT LOG

NAME:

GOALS:

DATE:

STATS:

WEIGHT:

EXERCISE:	SETS	REPS	WEIGHT	REST	SETS	REPS	WEIGHT	REST	SETS	REPS	WEIGHT	REST	SETS	REPS	WEIGHT	REST

CARDIO:	TIME	DIST.	INT.	PACE	TIME	DIST.	INT.	PACE	TIME	DIST.	INT.	PACE	TIME	DIST.	INT.	PACE

WORKOUT LOG

NAME:
GOALS:
DATE:
STATS:
WEIGHT:

EXERCISE:	SETS	REPS	WEIGHT	REST	SETS	REPS	WEIGHT	REST	SETS	REPS	WEIGHT	REST	SETS	REPS	WEIGHT	REST

CARDIO:	TIME	DIST.	INT.	PACE	TIME	DIST.	INT.	PACE	TIME	DIST.	INT.	PACE	TIME	DIST.	INT.	PACE

WORKOUT LOG

NAME:

GOALS:

DATE:

STATS:

WEIGHT:

EXERCISE:	SETS	REPS	WEIGHT	REST	SETS	REPS	WEIGHT	REST	SETS	REPS	WEIGHT	REST	SETS	REPS	WEIGHT	REST

CARDIO:	TIME	DIST.	INT.	PACE	TIME	DIST.	INT.	PACE	TIME	DIST.	INT.	PACE	TIME	DIST.	INT.	PACE

WORKOUT LOG

NAME: __________________________
GOALS: __________________________
DATE:
STATS:
WEIGHT:

EXERCISE:	SETS	REPS	WEIGHT	REST	SETS	REPS	WEIGHT	REST	SETS	REPS	WEIGHT	REST	SETS	REPS	WEIGHT	REST

CARDIO:	TIME	DIST.	INT.	PACE	TIME	DIST.	INT.	PACE	TIME	DIST.	INT.	PACE	TIME	DIST.	INT.	PACE

WORKOUT LOG

NAME:
GOALS:
DATE:
STATS:
WEIGHT:

EXERCISE:	SETS	REPS	WEIGHT	REST	SETS	REPS	WEIGHT	REST	SETS	REPS	WEIGHT	REST	SETS	REPS	WEIGHT	REST

CARDIO:	TIME	DIST.	INT.	PACE	TIME	DIST.	INT.	PACE	TIME	DIST.	INT.	PACE	TIME	DIST.	INT.	PACE

WORKOUT LOG

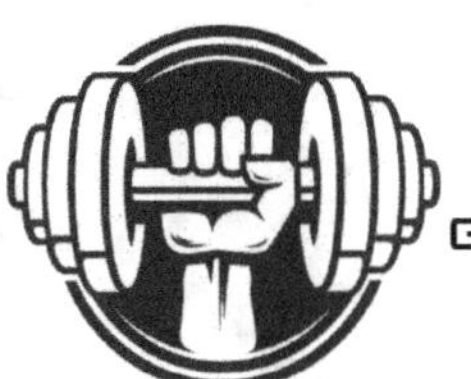

NAME: _______________________________

GOALS: _______________________________

DATE:

STATS:

WEIGHT:

EXERCISE:	SETS	REPS	WEIGHT	REST	SETS	REPS	WEIGHT	REST	SETS	REPS	WEIGHT	REST	SETS	REPS	WEIGHT	REST

CARDIO:	TIME	DIST.	INT.	PACE	TIME	DIST.	INT.	PACE	TIME	DIST.	INT.	PACE	TIME	DIST.	INT.	PACE

WORKOUT LOG

NAME: _______________________________

GOALS: _______________________________

DATE:

STATS:

WEIGHT:

EXERCISE:	SETS	REPS	WEIGHT	REST	SETS	REPS	WEIGHT	REST	SETS	REPS	WEIGHT	REST	SETS	REPS	WEIGHT	REST

CARDIO:	TIME	DIST.	INT.	PACE	TIME	DIST.	INT.	PACE	TIME	DIST.	INT.	PACE	TIME	DIST.	INT.	PACE

WORKOUT LOG

NAME:
GOALS:
DATE:
STATS:
WEIGHT:

EXERCISE:	SETS	REPS	WEIGHT	REST	SETS	REPS	WEIGHT	REST	SETS	REPS	WEIGHT	REST	SETS	REPS	WEIGHT	REST

CARDIO:	TIME	DIST.	INT.	PACE	TIME	DIST.	INT.	PACE	TIME	DIST.	INT.	PACE	TIME	DIST.	INT.	PACE

WORKOUT LOG

NAME:

GOALS:

DATE:

STATS:

WEIGHT:

EXERCISE:	SETS	REPS	WEIGHT	REST	SETS	REPS	WEIGHT	REST	SETS	REPS	WEIGHT	REST	SETS	REPS	WEIGHT	REST

CARDIO:	TIME	DIST.	INT.	PACE	TIME	DIST.	INT.	PACE	TIME	DIST.	INT.	PACE	TIME	DIST.	INT.	PACE

WORKOUT LOG

NAME:
GOALS:
DATE:
STATS:
WEIGHT:

EXERCISE:	SETS	REPS	WEIGHT	REST	SETS	REPS	WEIGHT	REST	SETS	REPS	WEIGHT	REST	SETS	REPS	WEIGHT	REST

CARDIO:	TIME	DIST.	INT.	PACE	TIME	DIST.	INT.	PACE	TIME	DIST.	INT.	PACE	TIME	DIST.	INT.	PACE

WORKOUT LOG

NAME:
GOALS:
DATE:
STATS:
WEIGHT:

EXERCISE:	SETS	REPS	WEIGHT	REST	SETS	REPS	WEIGHT	REST	SETS	REPS	WEIGHT	REST	SETS	REPS	WEIGHT	REST

CARDIO:	TIME	DIST.	INT.	PACE	TIME	DIST.	INT.	PACE	TIME	DIST.	INT.	PACE	TIME	DIST.	INT.	PACE

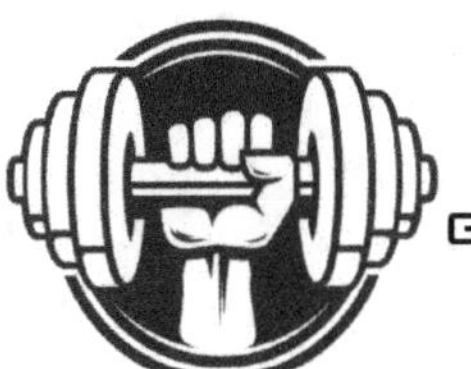

WORKOUT LOG

NAME: ______________________________
GOALS: ______________________________

DATE:
STATS:
WEIGHT:

EXERCISE:	SETS	REPS	WEIGHT	REST	SETS	REPS	WEIGHT	REST	SETS	REPS	WEIGHT	REST	SETS	REPS	WEIGHT	REST

CARDIO:	TIME	DIST.	INT.	PACE	TIME	DIST.	INT.	PACE	TIME	DIST.	INT.	PACE	TIME	DIST.	INT.	PACE

WORKOUT LOG

NAME:
GOALS:
DATE:
STATS:
WEIGHT:

EXERCISE:	SETS	REPS	WEIGHT	REST	SETS	REPS	WEIGHT	REST	SETS	REPS	WEIGHT	REST	SETS	REPS	WEIGHT	REST

CARDIO:	TIME	DIST.	INT.	PACE	TIME	DIST.	INT.	PACE	TIME	DIST.	INT.	PACE	TIME	DIST.	INT.	PACE

WORKOUT LOG

NAME:
GOALS:
DATE:
STATS:
WEIGHT:

EXERCISE:	SETS	REPS	WEIGHT	REST	SETS	REPS	WEIGHT	REST	SETS	REPS	WEIGHT	REST	SETS	REPS	WEIGHT	REST

CARDIO:	TIME	DIST.	INT.	PACE	TIME	DIST.	INT.	PACE	TIME	DIST.	INT.	PACE	TIME	DIST.	INT.	PACE

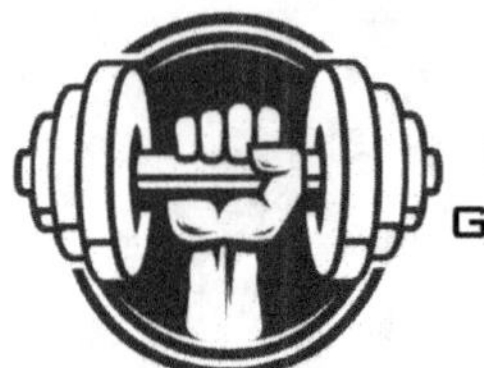

WORKOUT LOG

NAME:
GOALS:
DATE:
STATS:
WEIGHT:

EXERCISE:	SETS	REPS	WEIGHT	REST	SETS	REPS	WEIGHT	REST	SETS	REPS	WEIGHT	REST	SETS	REPS	WEIGHT	REST

CARDIO:	TIME	DIST.	INT.	PACE	TIME	DIST.	INT.	PACE	TIME	DIST.	INT.	PACE	TIME	DIST.	INT.	PACE

WORKOUT LOG

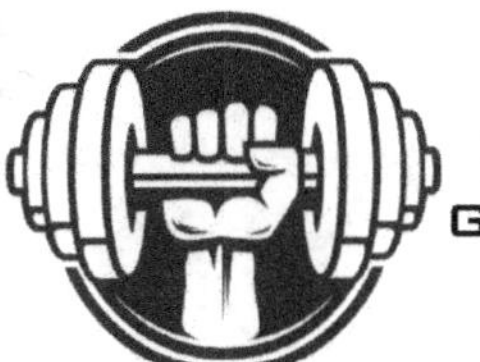

NAME:
GOALS:
DATE:
STATS:
WEIGHT:

EXERCISE:	SETS	REPS	WEIGHT	REST	SETS	REPS	WEIGHT	REST	SETS	REPS	WEIGHT	REST	SETS	REPS	WEIGHT	REST

CARDIO:	TIME	DIST.	INT.	PACE	TIME	DIST.	INT.	PACE	TIME	DIST.	INT.	PACE	TIME	DIST.	INT.	PACE

WORKOUT LOG

NAME:

GOALS:

DATE:

STATS:

WEIGHT:

EXERCISE:	SETS	REPS	WEIGHT	REST	SETS	REPS	WEIGHT	REST	SETS	REPS	WEIGHT	REST	SETS	REPS	WEIGHT	REST

CARDIO:	TIME	DIST.	INT.	PACE	TIME	DIST.	INT.	PACE	TIME	DIST.	INT.	PACE	TIME	DIST.	INT.	PACE

WORKOUT LOG

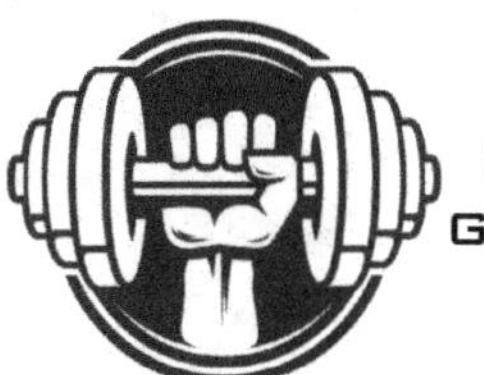

NAME:
GOALS:
DATE:
STATS:
WEIGHT:

EXERCISE:	SETS	REPS	WEIGHT	REST	SETS	REPS	WEIGHT	REST	SETS	REPS	WEIGHT	REST	SETS	REPS	WEIGHT	REST

CARDIO:	TIME	DIST.	INT.	PACE	TIME	DIST.	INT.	PACE	TIME	DIST.	INT.	PACE	TIME	DIST.	INT.	PACE

WORKOUT LOG

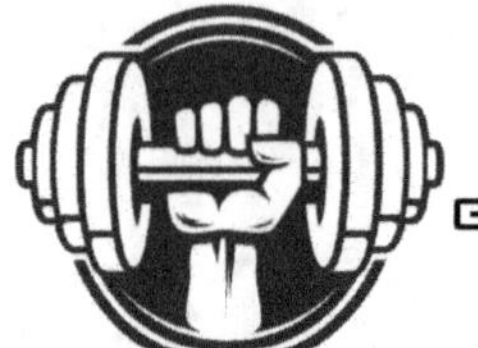

NAME:

GOALS:

DATE:

STATS:

WEIGHT:

EXERCISE:	SETS	REPS	WEIGHT	REST	SETS	REPS	WEIGHT	REST	SETS	REPS	WEIGHT	REST	SETS	REPS	WEIGHT	REST

CARDIO:	TIME	DIST.	INT.	PACE	TIME	DIST.	INT.	PACE	TIME	DIST.	INT.	PACE	TIME	DIST.	INT.	PACE

WORKOUT LOG

NAME:
GOALS:
DATE:
STATS:
WEIGHT:

EXERCISE:	SETS	REPS	WEIGHT	REST	SETS	REPS	WEIGHT	REST	SETS	REPS	WEIGHT	REST	SETS	REPS	WEIGHT	REST

CARDIO:	TIME	DIST.	INT.	PACE	TIME	DIST.	INT.	PACE	TIME	DIST.	INT.	PACE	TIME	DIST.	INT.	PACE

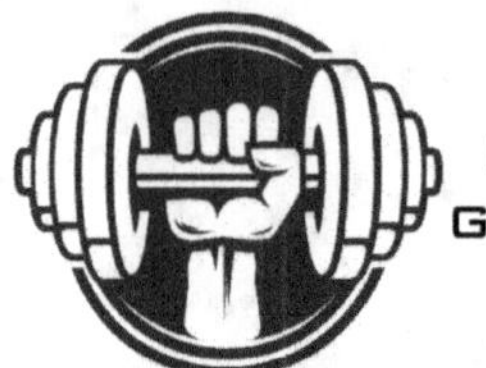

WORKOUT LOG

NAME: ________________________

GOALS: ________________________

DATE:

STATS:

WEIGHT:

EXERCISE:	SETS	REPS	WEIGHT	REST	SETS	REPS	WEIGHT	REST	SETS	REPS	WEIGHT	REST	SETS	REPS	WEIGHT	REST

CARDIO:	TIME	DIST.	INT.	PACE	TIME	DIST.	INT.	PACE	TIME	DIST.	INT.	PACE	TIME	DIST.	INT.	PACE

WORKOUT LOG

NAME:
GOALS:
DATE:
STATS:
WEIGHT:

EXERCISE:	SETS	REPS	WEIGHT	REST	SETS	REPS	WEIGHT	REST	SETS	REPS	WEIGHT	REST	SETS	REPS	WEIGHT	REST

CARDIO:	TIME	DIST.	INT.	PACE	TIME	DIST.	INT.	PACE	TIME	DIST.	INT.	PACE	TIME	DIST.	INT.	PACE

WORKOUT LOG

NAME:

GOALS:

DATE:

STATS:

WEIGHT:

EXERCISE:	SETS	REPS	WEIGHT	REST	SETS	REPS	WEIGHT	REST	SETS	REPS	WEIGHT	REST	SETS	REPS	WEIGHT	REST

CARDIO:	TIME	DIST.	INT.	PACE	TIME	DIST.	INT.	PACE	TIME	DIST.	INT.	PACE	TIME	DIST.	INT.	PACE

WORKOUT LOG

NAME:
GOALS:
DATE:
STATS:
WEIGHT:

EXERCISE:	SETS	REPS	WEIGHT	REST	SETS	REPS	WEIGHT	REST	SETS	REPS	WEIGHT	REST	SETS	REPS	WEIGHT	REST

CARDIO:	TIME	DIST.	INT.	PACE	TIME	DIST.	INT.	PACE	TIME	DIST.	INT.	PACE	TIME	DIST.	INT.	PACE

WORKOUT LOG

NAME:

GOALS:

DATE:

STATS:

WEIGHT:

EXERCISE:	SETS	REPS	WEIGHT	REST	SETS	REPS	WEIGHT	REST	SETS	REPS	WEIGHT	REST	SETS	REPS	WEIGHT	REST

CARDIO:	TIME	DIST.	INT.	PACE	TIME	DIST.	INT.	PACE	TIME	DIST.	INT.	PACE	TIME	DIST.	INT.	PACE

WORKOUT LOG

NAME:
GOALS:
DATE:
STATS:
WEIGHT:

EXERCISE:	SETS	REPS	WEIGHT	REST	SETS	REPS	WEIGHT	REST	SETS	REPS	WEIGHT	REST	SETS	REPS	WEIGHT	REST

CARDIO:	TIME	DIST.	INT.	PACE	TIME	DIST.	INT.	PACE	TIME	DIST.	INT.	PACE	TIME	DIST.	INT.	PACE

WORKOUT LOG

NAME:

GOALS:

DATE:

STATS:

WEIGHT:

EXERCISE:	SETS	REPS	WEIGHT	REST	SETS	REPS	WEIGHT	REST	SETS	REPS	WEIGHT	REST	SETS	REPS	WEIGHT	REST

CARDIO:	TIME	DIST.	INT.	PACE	TIME	DIST.	INT.	PACE	TIME	DIST.	INT.	PACE	TIME	DIST.	INT.	PACE

WORKOUT LOG

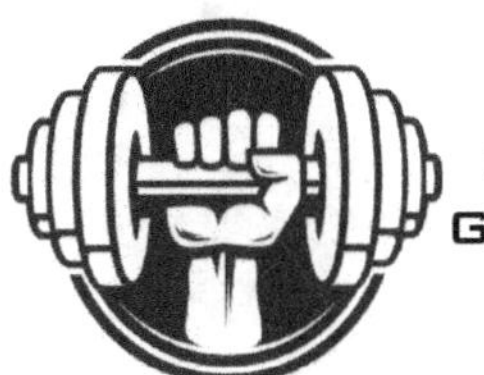

NAME:

GOALS:

DATE:

STATS:

WEIGHT:

EXERCISE:	SETS	REPS	WEIGHT	REST	SETS	REPS	WEIGHT	REST	SETS	REPS	WEIGHT	REST	SETS	REPS	WEIGHT	REST

CARDIO:	TIME	DIST.	INT.	PACE	TIME	DIST.	INT.	PACE	TIME	DIST.	INT.	PACE	TIME	DIST.	INT.	PACE

WORKOUT LOG

NAME: ______________________________

GOALS: ______________________________

DATE:

STATS:

WEIGHT:

EXERCISE:	SETS	REPS	WEIGHT	REST	SETS	REPS	WEIGHT	REST	SETS	REPS	WEIGHT	REST	SETS	REPS	WEIGHT	REST

CARDIO:	TIME	DIST.	INT.	PACE	TIME	DIST.	INT.	PACE	TIME	DIST.	INT.	PACE	TIME	DIST.	INT.	PACE

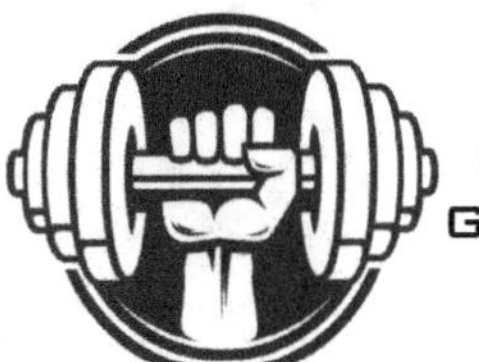

WORKOUT LOG

NAME:

GOALS:

DATE:

STATS:

WEIGHT:

EXERCISE:	SETS	REPS	WEIGHT	REST	SETS	REPS	WEIGHT	REST	SETS	REPS	WEIGHT	REST	SETS	REPS	WEIGHT	REST

CARDIO:	TIME	DIST.	INT.	PACE	TIME	DIST.	INT.	PACE	TIME	DIST.	INT.	PACE	TIME	DIST.	INT.	PACE

WORKOUT LOG

NAME:
GOALS:
DATE:
STATS:
WEIGHT:

EXERCISE:	SETS	REPS	WEIGHT	REST	SETS	REPS	WEIGHT	REST	SETS	REPS	WEIGHT	REST	SETS	REPS	WEIGHT	REST

CARDIO:	TIME	DIST.	INT.	PACE	TIME	DIST.	INT.	PACE	TIME	DIST.	INT.	PACE	TIME	DIST.	INT.	PACE

WORKOUT LOG

NAME: ___________________________

GOALS: ___________________________

DATE:

STATS:

WEIGHT:

EXERCISE:	SETS	REPS	WEIGHT	REST	SETS	REPS	WEIGHT	REST	SETS	REPS	WEIGHT	REST	SETS	REPS	WEIGHT	REST

CARDIO:	TIME	DIST.	INT.	PACE	TIME	DIST.	INT.	PACE	TIME	DIST.	INT.	PACE	TIME	DIST.	INT.	PACE

WORKOUT LOG

NAME:

GOALS:

DATE:

STATS:

WEIGHT:

EXERCISE:	SETS	REPS	WEIGHT	REST	SETS	REPS	WEIGHT	REST	SETS	REPS	WEIGHT	REST	SETS	REPS	WEIGHT	REST

CARDIO:	TIME	DIST.	INT.	PACE	TIME	DIST.	INT.	PACE	TIME	DIST.	INT.	PACE	TIME	DIST.	INT.	PACE

www.ingramcontent.com/pod-product-compliance
Lightning Source LLC
Chambersburg PA
CBHW070737250726
48662CB00004B/1568